The Human Dietary Conspiracy

How Government Subsidizes Your Early Death

By

Alice Dee

DEDICATION

This book is gratefully dedicated to the love of my life.

ACKNOWLEDGEMENTS

I wish to acknowledge the inspiration of my dear friends who have been able to look behind the veil of the mainstream media and traditional dietary patterns to illuminate the truths every human should know to live a longer and healthier life well into retirement.

TABLE OF CONTENTS

PREFACE

Dear Readers,

Welcome to a book intended to awaken your understanding of the hidden forces shaping your health and well-being. In this book, we will explore the "Human Dietary Conspiracy," a web of mainstream media-propagated misinformation, manipulated government food policies, and vested corporate interests that silently undermine our health and shorten our lifespans.

We'll delve into the murky depths of subsidized processed foods, unveiling the hidden sugar, salt and other additives that fuel an addiction epidemic and contribute to a multitude of chronic diseases. We'll expose the myths surrounding bread and wheat, revealing the truth behind their impact on our bodies, and guide you through navigating this complex food landscape.

This book also sheds light on the elusive truth about saturated fats, disentangling the hype from the facts and empowering you to make informed dietary choices based on solid scientific evidence. We'll also embrace the wisdom of our ancestors and explore the transformative power of a raw whole foods diet in unlocking a new dimension of health and vitality.

Unraveling the processed food labyrinth, you'll learn to decipher the cryptic language of food labels and create a healthy haven within your own kitchen. We'll also dismantle the meat myth, exposing the environmental, health and ethical costs of animal agriculture and presenting healthier, more sustainable alternatives.

Throughout this book, I aim to arm you with practical tools and resources to empower you to reclaim control of your present and future health. You'll discover the secrets of a thriving and long-lasting retirement, free from the burden of chronic illnesses.

We also need to cultivate a sense of community, supporting each other as we rise up against the prevailing dietary deception propaganda and forge a brighter future for ourselves and generations to come.

This book is not just about changing your diet; it's about changing the world, its future, and your health. It's a call to action, a clarion call to break free from the shackles of misinformation and embrace a new paradigm of health and well-being. Let us embark on this transformative path together, one delicious and healthy bite at a time.

Prepare to be empowered. Prepare to be inspired. Prepare to reclaim your health, extend your life well into retirement, and rewrite the dietary narrative for a future filled with vitality, longevity, and sustainable practices.

Throughout these pages, you'll find a fusion of scientific rigor with practical tips that are all based on my genuine passion for promoting optimal health in my readers. My hope is that this book serves as a guide for you, sparking thoughtful reflection on the choices we all make in the kitchen and paving your way toward a lifestyle that not only supports but propels you toward your highest health potential.

Thank you for bravely embarking on this path with me into the shady details of the Human Dietary Conspiracy. May your explorations herein illuminate your understanding of the ideal diet for humanity and remain a catalyst for positive change in your life.

To your health!

Alice Dee

THE HUMAN DIETARY CONSPIRACY

INTRODUCTION

The human body is a magnificent machine, built to endure for up to 120 years. Yet, in today's world, we face a paradox: while our life expectancy is increasing, we're dying younger than ever before.

This grim reality isn't simply a matter of fate; it's the product of a complex web of misinformation, manipulation, and government policies that prioritize profit over public health. In this book, we'll expose the shocking truth behind the "Human Dietary Conspiracy," revealing how the government's hidden hand is literally shortening your life.

Imagine a world where the foods you crave most are not just delicious, but also designed to be addictive and ultimately harmful. This isn't science fiction; it's the reality we face every day. The food industry, with its multi-billion dollar marketing campaigns and powerful lobbying forces, has infiltrated our kitchens and our minds, convincing us that processed, sugar-laden products are essential for happiness and well-being.

Unfortunately, behind the glossy packaging and sugary promises lies a truth far more sinister. These processed foods, heavily subsidized by the government, are laden with hidden dangers, fueling an epidemic of chronic diseases that shorten lifespans and cripple healthcare systems.

The government's role in this conspiracy is undeniable. Billions of dollars are funneled each year into supporting the animal agriculture and processed food industries through a labyrinthine system of price supports, tax breaks, and other financial incentives.

These subsidies, intended to ensure food security, have ironically or possibly intentionally created a perverse situation where unhealthy foods are readily available and affordable, while nutritious options often remain out of reach for many. This deliberate manipulation of the food system makes paying out social security benefits to retirees more feasible and prioritizes profit over public health, sacrificing our well-being for the sake of a few powerful corporations.

The consequences of this conspiracy are devastating. Chronic diseases like heart disease, diabetes, and cancer are on the rise, plaguing individuals and families with physical and financial hardship.

These diseases don't just impact our quality of life; they shorten lifespans, leading to premature deaths that could have been prevented. This not only causes immense personal grief but also creates a significant burden on society as a whole, straining healthcare systems and jeopardizing the future of critical programs like Social Security.

But this is not a story of hopelessness. Within these pages, we'll not only expose the truth about the Human Dietary Conspiracy, but also equip you with the knowledge and tools to break free from its grip.

You'll discover the science behind healthy eating, learn how to decipher misleading food labels, and gain practical tips for creating a diet rich in whole, nutritious foods. We'll explore alternative food systems that prioritize sustainability and ethical practices, empowering you to make conscious choices for your health and the planet.

This book is not just a call to action; it's a call to revolution. It's time to reclaim control of our health and our food choices. By raising awareness, challenging the status quo, and demanding change, we can create a healthier future for ourselves and generations to come.

Join me on this journey now as we expose the truth, break the chains of the dietary conspiracy, and build a world where food nourishes our bodies, extends our lifespan, and empowers our lives.

CHAPTER 1: THE LONGEVITY LOOPHOLE: SOCIAL SECURITY AND FOOD SUBSIDIES COLLIDE

The United States and many other industrialized nations now stand at a crossroads. As the population ages and retires, the question of how to support a growing number of retirees becomes increasingly urgent.

Social Security, the bedrock of financial security for countless Americans, faces the specter of depletion, casting a shadow over the future of millions. At the heart of this issue lies a complex web of economic incentives, dietary trends, and public health concerns.

One cannot ignore the rising cost of Social Security. With each passing year, the discrepancy between the program's income and expenditure widens.

This demographic shift, fueled by increasing life expectancy and declining birth rates, creates a scenario where the system's ability to fulfill its promises becomes increasingly precarious. Projections paint a grim picture, with the possibility of Social Security Trust Funds running dry as early as 2034.

The political landscape surrounding potential solutions is fraught with contention. Proposals to raise the retirement age, reduce benefits, or introduce alternative funding mechanisms often encounter fierce resistance from various stakeholders. The debate remains mired in a cycle of partisan gridlock, offering little in the way of concrete solutions.

Deadly Government Food Subsides

Even as political discourse stalls on the retirement issue, another factor quietly plays a significant role in the equation: the government's extensive support of the animal agriculture and processed food industries. Through a labyrinthine network of price supports, tax breaks, and other financial instruments, billions of taxpayer dollars are funneled into these industries each year.

The ostensible purpose of these subsidies is to bolster agricultural production and ensure food security. However, they come at a hidden cost – the promotion of unhealthy dietary habits. The animal foods rendered readily available and affordable through this system are often laden with saturated fat, while processed foods abound in sodium and added sugars. The end result is that this highly questionable government food policy contributes to the rising tide of chronic diseases like heart disease, stroke, obesity, high blood pressure, high cholesterol, type II diabetes, and cancer.

Furthermore, the very foods that sustain a healthy human life – raw fruits, greens, grains, legumes, nuts and seeds – are not subsidized at all and so cost more in comparison to unhealthy food choices that the government subsidies push upon the price-sensitive public. Even government food banks ostensibly intended to feed the poor provide a dearth of healthy raw plant foods, instead offering harmful animal products and canned foods devoid of much of their original nutritional value.

The Perverse Cycle of Unhealthy Subsidies

Governments deliberately subsidizing remarkably unhealthy foods ultimately create a perverse cycle. The very system designed to secure the future of Social Security and provide food for less wealthy Americans inadvertently fuels their joint demise.

By actively encouraging the consumption of unhealthy foods among the price-sensitive public by making them cheaper, the government actively contributes to shortening its citizens' lifespans that in turn eases its obligation to pay them retirement benefits.

Unfortunately, this covert policy not only causes early deaths, but it can also lead to higher healthcare costs among the sickening population which can further strain the retirement program's financial resources. This is a self-inflicted wound, one that undermines the very foundation of economic stability and health for millions of Americans.

How Government Food Policies Need to Change

The path forward to healthier government food policies demands a radical shift in policy and priorities. We must move beyond the antiquated notion of supporting unhealthy food systems and embrace a future where public health and financial sustainability are inextricably linked. This requires:

- Reforming the subsidy system: Diverting government support from animal agriculture and processed foods towards sustainable, plant-based agricultural practices that prioritize the production of healthy and nutritious options.

- Investing in public health initiatives: Empowering individuals to make informed dietary choices through education and awareness campaigns, while ensuring access to affordable, nutritious food across all communities.

- Creating a regulatory framework: Implementing policies that disincentivize the production and consumption of unhealthy foods, while fostering innovation and development in the plant-based food sector.

These steps are not merely economic considerations; they are investments in the nation's health and future. By embracing a holistic approach that addresses the root causes of rising healthcare costs and promotes healthy lifestyles, we can ensure a more secure Social Security system and a brighter future for generations to come.

The choice before us is clear. We can continue on the current path, perpetuating a system that undermines our collective well-being and financial stability. Or, we can choose a different route, one that prioritizes health, sustainability, and the long-term prosperity of our nation.

The future of Social Security, and ultimately, the well-being of millions of Americans, rests on the decisions we make today. We must act now to break the cycle of early deaths and financial instability, paving the way for a healthier and more secure future for all.

CHAPTER 2: A SPOONFUL OF SUGAR MAKES THE GOVERNMENT GO DOWN

The human palate is a fickle beast. It craves sweetness, saltiness, and fat, often prioritizing pleasure over nutrition. This inherent biological inclination, coupled with the relentless marketing prowess of the food industry, has led to a societal shift towards processed, convenient foods. This seemingly innocuous preference has, however, yielded a devastating consequence: a decline in our collective health.

This chapter delves into the heart of this issue, exploring the rise of processed foods and its impact on our health, the insidious influence of the Big Food lobby, and the government's role in perpetuating this unhealthy and unsustainable food system.

The Rise of Processed Foods and the Decline of Health

The modern world demands convenience. We juggle careers, families, and personal lives, leaving little time for elaborate meals. This has fueled the rise of processed food, offering a quick and seemingly easy solution. These readily available options, however, come at a hidden cost.

Processed foods are typically devoid of vital nutrients and fiber, while simultaneously laden with unhealthy ingredients like added sugars, unhealthy fats, and excessive sodium. These components, designed to tantalize taste buds and promote addiction, contribute to a cascade of chronic diseases.

Excess sugar, often hidden in seemingly healthy products, wreaks havoc on our metabolic health. It disrupts insulin sensitivity, leading to elevated blood sugar levels and ultimately increasing the risk of diabetes. Unhealthy fats, particularly saturated and trans fats, contribute to heart disease and stroke, the leading causes of death globally. Sodium, another ubiquitous ingredient in processed foods, elevates blood pressure, placing further strain on our cardiovascular systems.

The consequences of this dietary shift are evident in our communities. Obesity rates are soaring, particularly among children and adolescents, paving the way for a future burdened by chronic illnesses. This epidemic not only impacts individual lives but also strains healthcare systems, putting a significant financial burden on society.

The Big Food Lobby's Grip on Policy

The Big Food industry, a multi-billion dollar behemoth, wields significant power over our food system. Through aggressive marketing campaigns and relentless lobbying efforts, they have successfully manipulated public perception and influenced government policies.

Their marketing campaigns are designed to be irresistible, targeting children and adults alike. Colorful packaging, cartoon characters, and manipulative advertising create a false image of health and happiness associated with their products. This potent marketing often overshadows the nutritional realities, leading to impulsive choices and unhealthy dietary habits.

But the influence extends beyond marketing. The Big Food lobby has a substantial presence in Washington, influencing food policy and legislation to favor their interests. They advocate for subsidies that support the production of unhealthy ingredients and oppose policies that promote healthy eating initiatives. This influence allows them to maintain the status quo, prioritizing profit over public health.

How Subsidies Make Unhealthy Foods Cheap and Healthy Food Expensive

One of the most insidious aspects of this conspiracy is the government's role in subsidizing the production of unhealthy foods. Through a complex system of price supports, tax breaks, and other financial incentives, the government unknowingly fuels the consumption of processed food.

These subsidies artificially lower the cost of unhealthy ingredients, making them readily available and affordable, particularly for low-income families. Conversely, healthy options like fresh produce, whole grains, and lean protein remain relatively expensive, creating a significant disparity in access to nutritious food.

This system effectively creates a two-tiered food system, one that promotes unhealthy choices for the majority while making the healthy option inaccessible. This not only perpetuates the cycle of chronic diseases but also exacerbates existing social inequalities.

The Human Dietary Conspiracy is a complex web of manipulation, misinformation, and misplaced priorities. By understanding the rise of processed foods, the influence of the Big Food lobby, and the government's role in subsidizing unhealthy choices, we begin to see the truth behind this insidious system. Only by dismantling this conspiracy can we create a food system that prioritizes health, sustainability, and the well-being of all.

CHAPTER 3: THE SUGAR TRAP: HOW YOUR SWEET TOOTH IS KILLING YOU

Sugar, that seemingly innocent white powder, holds a dark secret. It is not just a flavor enhancer; it is a potent addictive substance that wreaks havoc on our bodies, minds, and ultimately, our lives.

This chapter delves into the science behind sugar addiction, exposing the hidden sugars lurking in unexpected places, and exploring the potentially harmful consequences of artificial sweeteners.

The Science Behind Sugar Addiction

Sugar, specifically sucrose, triggers the release of dopamine, a neurotransmitter associated with pleasure and reward. This surge of dopamine creates a sense of euphoria, reinforcing the desire for more sugar.

Over time, repeated exposure to sugar leads to changes in the brain, similar to those observed in addiction to drugs like cocaine. The brain becomes desensitized to dopamine, requiring increasingly larger doses of sugar to achieve the same pleasurable effect.

A 2013 study published in the journal Nature Neuroscience by Princeton University researchers revealed striking similarities in the brain activity of sugar-addicted rats and humans addicted to drugs like cocaine. This research provides compelling evidence that sugar addiction is a legitimate neurological condition, demanding serious attention and intervention.

The addictive nature of sugar is further amplified by its influence on another key neurotransmitter, serotonin. Serotonin plays a vital role in regulating mood, appetite, and sleep.

When serotonin levels are low, we experience cravings for sugary treats, seeking the temporary boost in mood and energy that sugar provides.

However, this initial uplift is followed by a crash, leaving us feeling tired, irritable, and craving more sugar. This creates a vicious cycle that can be difficult to break.

Hidden Sugars in Unexpected Places

The sugar trap is particularly insidious because sugar is often hidden in seemingly healthy foods. Food manufacturers cleverly disguise sugar under various names, making it difficult for consumers to make informed choices.

Common aliases include high-fructose corn syrup, sucrose, dextrose, and maltose, to name just a few. These hidden sugars are omnipresent, lurking in everything from breakfast cereals and yogurt to salad dressings and pasta sauces.

A 2012 study published in the Journal of the American Medical Association (JAMA) found that added sugars constitute a staggering 17% of the average American's daily calorie intake. This alarming statistic highlights the extent to which sugar has infiltrated our food supply, contributing to an epidemic of obesity, diabetes, and other chronic diseases.

One of the most deceptive tactics employed by food manufacturers is the use of "natural" sweeteners like honey and agave nectar. While these may sound healthier than refined sugar, their chemical composition is essentially the same. They contain roughly the same amount of fructose, a potent sugar linked to a range of health problems.

The Real Cost of Artificial Sweeteners

In an effort to curb sugar intake and its associated health risks, many individuals turn to artificial sweeteners. Aspartame, sucralose, and saccharin are the most common culprits, marketed as guilt-free alternatives to sugar. However, the long-term health effects of these artificial sweeteners remain controversial and warrant further investigation.

A 2017 meta-analysis published in the journal PLOS Medicine analyzed 11 studies investigating the relationship between artificial sweetener consumption and cancer risk. The researchers found a statistically significant association between consuming artificial sweeteners and an increased risk of cancer, particularly hematological malignancies and certain types of brain tumors.

Furthermore, artificial sweeteners have been linked to a range of other health concerns, including:

- Metabolic syndrome: A cluster of risk factors that increase the risk of cardiovascular disease and diabetes.

- Cognitive decline: Studies suggest that artificial sweeteners may impair memory and learning, particularly in older adults.

- Gut microbiome disruption: Artificial sweeteners may alter the composition of gut bacteria, potentially leading to digestive issues and other health problems.

Breaking the Cycle

The good news is that we can break free from the sugar trap by taking control of our food choices and adopting a more mindful approach to eating. Here are some practical steps to achieve this:

- **Read food labels carefully:** Pay close attention to the ingredients list and avoid products that contain added sugars, regardless of the name they are listed under. Many seemingly healthy foods like yogurt and salad dressings can contain surprisingly high amounts of sugar. Use resources like the Food and Drug Administration's website to learn about different sugar aliases and how to identify them on food labels.

- **Choose whole foods over processed foods:** Opt for fresh fruits, vegetables, whole grains, and lean protein sources over packaged foods that are typically laden with sugar and other unhealthy ingredients. Whole foods provide essential nutrients and fiber, helping you feel full and satisfied, reducing cravings for sugary treats.

- **Limit sugary drinks:** Ditch the soda, fruit juices, and sugary coffee drinks and opt for water, unsweetened tea, or black coffee instead. Liquid calories add up quickly, and sugary drinks contribute significantly to our daily sugar intake. Choosing water or unsweetened beverages helps you stay hydrated and avoid unnecessary sugar consumption.

- **Cook more meals at home:** This gives you greater control over the ingredients in your food and allows you to avoid hidden sugars.

Cooking at home allows you to use fresh, whole ingredients and customize recipes to your preferences. You can also experiment with healthier cooking methods, like grilling, baking, and steaming, to avoid adding unnecessary fats and sugars.

- **Seek support:** Talk to a registered dietitian or nutritionist for personalized guidance on developing a healthy eating plan that meets your individual needs and preferences. These professionals can provide valuable advice on managing sugar cravings, creating balanced meals, and navigating the complexities of food labels and healthy eating.

Cultivating a Mindful Approach

Beyond dietary changes, cultivating a mindful approach to eating plays a key role in breaking free from the sugar trap. This involves:

- **Paying attention to hunger and fullness cues:** Learn to distinguish between true hunger and emotional or boredom-induced cravings. Eat only when you're physically hungry and stop when you feel comfortably full, avoiding overindulgence.

- **Slowing down and savoring your food:** Chew your food thoroughly and enjoy the taste and texture of each bite. This helps with mindful eating and can increase satiety, reducing the urge to overeat.

- **Identifying and managing triggers:** Pay attention to situations or emotions that trigger sugar cravings. Stress, boredom, and social situations can all be triggers. Develop healthy coping mechanisms to manage these triggers, such as exercise, relaxation techniques, or engaging in activities you enjoy.

- **Focusing on long-term health benefits:** Remind yourself of the positive outcomes of breaking free from the sugar trap. This can include increased energy levels, improved mood, weight management, and a reduced risk of chronic diseases.

Building a Sustainable Lifestyle

Breaking free from the sugar trap is not just about making temporary changes; it's about building a sustainable lifestyle that supports your health and well-being. Here are some key steps:

- **Set realistic goals:** Start with small, achievable goals and gradually work your way towards bigger changes. Attempting drastic changes overnight is often unsustainable and can lead to discouragement.

- **Celebrate small victories:** Acknowledge and celebrate your progress, no matter how small. This helps stay motivated and reinforces positive behaviors.

- **Find support:** Surround yourself with friends and family who share your health and dietary goals and encourage you on your path. Join a support group or online community to connect with others who are also working to break free from the sugar trap.

- **Be patient and kind to yourself:** Change takes time and effort. Don't be discouraged by setbacks. Instead, learn from them and recommit yourself to your goals. Remember, progress over perfection is key.

By taking control of your food choices, practicing mindfulness, and building a sustainable lifestyle, you can break free from the sugar trap and reclaim control of your health and well-being.

Remember, you are not alone in this process. There are countless resources available and people willing to lend you support to help you along the way. So, take the first step today and embark on the path towards a healthier and happier you.

CHAPTER 4: THE GRAIN GAME: WHY BREAD IS THE ENEMY OF YOUR HEALTH

The fragrant aroma of freshly baked bread has for millennia lured us in, symbolizing comfort, nourishment, and the bounty of the harvest. Yet, the simple loaf that once sustained our ancestors has morphed into a potential threat to our health in the modern age.

This transformation lies at the heart of the industrialization of wheat production, a process that has traded nutrition for efficiency and convenience, leaving us with a refined grain that may be jeopardizing our well-being.

The Rise of Industrial Wheat: A Sacrifice of Health for Yield

The 20th century witnessed a dramatic shift in how wheat was cultivated and processed. In the pursuit of higher yields and resistance to disease, traditional wheat varieties were cast aside in favor of genetically engineered hybrids. While these new strains promised bountiful harvests and economic prosperity, they came at a cost.

The focus on yield led to a significant increase in the gluten content of wheat, a protein responsible for the doughy texture of bread. Research published in the journal "Nature" in 2012 found that modern wheat varieties contain up to 70% more gluten than their ancient counterparts. This increase has been linked to a rise in gluten-related disorders, including celiac disease and gluten sensitivity, affecting millions worldwide.

Furthermore, the industrial processing of wheat strips the grain of its bran and germ, the parts containing the majority of its fiber, vitamins, and minerals. This results in "refined" wheat flour, which is then used to produce the vast majority of bread, pasta, and other baked goods found on supermarket shelves. These products, often laden with added sugars, unhealthy fats, and artificial ingredients, further exacerbate the negative health impacts of refined wheat.

A 2017 study published in the "Journal of the American Medical Association" found a strong correlation between the consumption of refined grains and an increased risk of obesity, type 2 diabetes, and heart disease. This research highlights the devastating impact of industrial wheat on our health, contributing to the growing epidemic of chronic diseases.

The Whole Wheat Myth: A Misleading Label

In response to growing concerns about the health implications of refined wheat, whole wheat bread emerged as a seemingly healthy alternative. However, the perception of whole wheat bread as a nutritional powerhouse may be misleading. While it retains some of the bran and germ, the majority of the grain is still refined, losing valuable nutrients in the process.

Additionally, many commercially produced whole wheat breads contain significant amounts of added sugars and unhealthy fats. A 2015 study by the Environmental Working Group found that 84% of whole wheat bread samples contained added sugar, with some containing as much sugar as a slice of cake. These hidden sugars negate the potential health benefits of whole wheat and contribute to excessive calorie intake.

For those seeking a truly healthy bread option, the best approach is to choose sprouted grain breads or bake with whole wheat flour at home. Sprouted grains offer increased digestibility and nutrient bioavailability, while baking at home allows for control over ingredients and ensures the absence of added sugars and unhealthy fats.

Gluten Sensitivity and Celiac Disease: A Growing Epidemic

The rise of industrial wheat has coincided with a significant increase in gluten sensitivity and celiac disease. Celiac disease is a serious autoimmune disorder triggered by gluten consumption, leading to damage to the small intestine and various health problems, including malnutrition, anemia, and fatigue.

A 2017 study published in the journal "Gastroenterology" estimated that 1 in 133 Americans suffer from celiac disease, representing a significant rise from previous estimates. This increase is believed to be linked to the increased gluten content of modern wheat and the ubiquitous presence of gluten in processed foods.

Gluten sensitivity, although not as severe as celiac disease, still causes unpleasant symptoms like bloating, diarrhea, and fatigue in affected individuals. A 2012 study by the University of Maryland found that nearly 6% of the population experiences gluten sensitivity, highlighting the widespread prevalence of this condition.

For individuals with gluten sensitivity or celiac disease, avoiding all gluten-containing products, including wheat, barley, and rye, is essential for maintaining good health and managing symptoms. This requires careful attention to food labels and opting for naturally gluten-free alternatives like quinoa, oats, and brown rice.

Beyond Bread: The Hidden Reach of Industrial Wheat

The impact of industrial wheat extends far beyond the realm of bread. Wheat is a hidden ingredient found in a vast array of processed foods, from breakfast cereals and crackers to sauces and condiments. This ubiquitous presence makes it even more challenging to avoid gluten and other potentially detrimental components of wheat.

A 2019 study by the Center for Science in the Public Interest found that wheat is present in over 80% of processed foods in supermarkets. This means that even seemingly innocuous products like salad dressings, ice cream, and even some medications may contain hidden wheat ingredients.

This widespread use of wheat highlights the need for consumers to become label-reading detectives. Carefully scrutinizing ingredient lists and prioritizing whole, unprocessed foods is crucial for minimizing exposure to refined wheat and its associated health risks.

Reclaiming Control: A Guide to Navigating the Wheat Maze

In the face of the pervasive presence of industrial wheat, individuals seeking to optimize their health have several strategies at their disposal.

- Embrace whole grains: Opt for naturally gluten-free whole grains like quinoa, brown rice, and buckwheat instead of refined wheat products. These grains provide complex carbohydrates, fiber, and essential nutrients for optimal health.

- Read labels meticulously: Pay close attention to ingredient lists and learn to recognize hidden wheat aliases like "wheat flour," "wheat starch," and "hydrolyzed wheat protein." Choose products that are labeled "gluten-free" or use certified gluten-free ingredients.

- Prepare meals at home: Cooking at home allows you to control the ingredients in your food and avoid hidden wheat sources. Experiment with gluten-free recipes and discover the joy of creating delicious and nutritious meals.

- Diversify your dietary sources: Explore alternative sources of carbohydrates like fruits, vegetables, and legumes. These provide complex carbohydrates, fiber, and a variety of essential vitamins and minerals, promoting a balanced and nutritious diet.

- Seek professional guidance: Consult with a registered dietitian or nutritionist for personalized guidance on navigating the complexities of food labels and developing a healthy eating plan that addresses your specific needs and preferences.

By embracing these strategies, individuals can reclaim control of their health and navigate the wheat maze with greater awareness and confidence. This transition towards a wheat-free lifestyle is not just about avoiding a single ingredient; it's about embracing a whole new way of eating, one that prioritizes whole, unprocessed foods and empowers us to nourish our bodies with the fuel they need to thrive.

Remember, the key to a healthy and fulfilling life lies in the choices we make each day. By making informed decisions about the food we consume, we can unlock a world of vibrant health and well-being, free from the grip of our modern-day wheat adversary.

CHAPTER 5: THE TRUTH ABOUT SATURATED FATS

The world of nutrition is a complex and ever-evolving landscape, with pronouncements about the "good" and "bad" food choices constantly shifting.

Saturated fats, correctly demonized as the dietary villains responsible for a plethora of health problems, now find themselves in a perplexing state of ambiguity, with their true negative impact on our well-being shrouded in a haze of misleading information.

This chapter delves into the science behind saturated fats, exploring their potential health risks, as well as the benefits of consuming moderate amounts of polyunsaturated fats. It ultimately aims to provide readers with the tools to navigate the maze of fat-related health claims and make better-informed dietary decisions.

Unmasking the Molecule: Understanding Saturated Fats

Before venturing into the debate surrounding saturated fats, it is essential to understand their basic composition. Unlike their unsaturated counterparts, which boast double bonds in their fatty acid chains, saturated fats lack these bonds, resulting in a straighter, more stable structure.

This structural difference manifests in their physical properties, making them solid at room temperature and contributing to the texture of many animal-derived foods.

The Impact of Saturated Fats on Cholesterol

The primary concern surrounding saturated fats lies in their interaction with cholesterol. When ingested, they raise levels of "bad" LDL cholesterol, a major player in the development of atherosclerosis, a condition characterized by the buildup of plaque in arteries.

This plaque restricts blood flow, ultimately greatly increasing the risk of heart disease and stroke, as well as other serious chronic diseases like arthritis and dementia.

However, it is important to note that some individuals respond differently to dietary saturated fat intake. Genetic predispositions and other factors can influence how efficiently the body metabolizes cholesterol, leading to varying responses across individuals.

Beyond Heart Disease: Exploring the Broader Health Implications

The negative impact of saturated fats extends beyond heart health. Research suggests potential links between their consumption and various chronic diseases, including:

- **Inflammation and chronic disease:** Saturated fats possess pro-inflammatory properties, contributing to the chronic inflammation associated with conditions like type 2 diabetes, certain cancers, and autoimmune disorders.

- **Insulin resistance and type 2 diabetes:** Excessive saturated fat intake can lead to insulin resistance, a condition where cells become less responsive to the hormone insulin, a key player in regulating blood sugar levels. This paves the way for the development of type 2 diabetes.

- **Cognitive decline and Alzheimer's disease:** Emerging research suggests a potential association between high saturated fat intake and cognitive decline, including an increased risk of developing Alzheimer's disease. While the exact mechanisms remain under investigation, saturated fats (and the animal proteins they typically come with) may contribute to the accumulation of harmful proteins in the brain associated with Alzheimer's disease, as well as clogging arteries that feed the brain and causing vascular dementia.

Beyond the Hype: Exploring Healthier Fat Sources

While reducing saturated fat intake is definitely important for promoting overall well-being, it is equally important to embrace moderate amounts of healthier alternatives with the overall goal of keeping total dietary fat content below the 20% level of total calories consumed.

Unsaturated fats from plants, categorized as monounsaturated and polyunsaturated, offer numerous health benefits including:

- **Monounsaturated fats:** Found in olive oil, avocados, and nuts, these fats improve heart health by lowering LDL cholesterol and raising HDL ("good") cholesterol levels.

- **Polyunsaturated fats:** These fats are further classified as omega-3 and omega-6 fatty acids. The omega 3 fatty acids are especially essential for brain function, cell growth, and reducing inflammation. Algal oil from marine algae provides the helpful EPA and DHA omega-3s, while flaxseeds, walnuts, and chia seeds are rich in Alpha Linoleic Acid that helps form omega-3s.

Navigating the Supermarket Maze: Deciphering Food Labels and Managing Your Diet

Making informed choices about dietary fat requires careful navigation of food labels and thoughtful management of your overall diet. Here are some key strategies:

- **Understanding food labels:** Pay close attention to the "Total Fat," "Saturated Fat," and "Unsaturated Fat" sections on the Nutrition Facts panel. Scrutinize the ingredient list to identify hidden sources of saturated fat that include all animal derived fats like butter, cheese, lard, milk and beef fat, as well as plant-derived saturated fats like partially hydrogenated oils, hydrogenated vegetable oil, coconut oil and palm oil.

- **Identifying hidden sources:** Be mindful of processed foods like baked goods, snack foods, and frozen meals, which often harbor hidden saturated fats. Prioritize whole, unprocessed foods whenever possible.

- **Building a balanced diet:** Focus on a diet rich in fruits, leafy greens and other vegetables, whole grains, legumes, nuts and seeds. This approach ensures a balanced intake of essential nutrients and minimizes exposure to harmful saturated fats.

Embracing a Holistic Approach: Beyond Diet and Towards Optimal Health

Reducing saturated fat intake is just one piece of the puzzle in achieving optimal health. A comprehensive approach involves incorporating other lifestyle changes:

Engaging in regular physical activity strengthens the heart, improves blood flow, and helps maintain a healthy weight, all contributing to reducing the risk of heart disease and other chronic conditions.

Effective stress management is important since chronic stress can negatively impact health. Techniques like meditation and yoga can help manage stress, lower blood pressure, reduce inflammation, and improve overall well-being. These practices can also promote better sleep quality, which is crucial for physical and mental health.

Taking Control of Your Health and Making Sustainable Choices

By making informed dietary choices, incorporating healthy lifestyle habits, and engaging in mindful practices, you can take control of your health and reduce your risk of chronic diseases.

Remember, small, sustainable changes implemented over time can have a significant impact on your overall well-being. Start small, experiment with different healthy options, and find what works best for you.

Conclusion: A Process of Continuous Learning and Growth

The path towards optimal health and a balanced relationship with food is a continuous process of learning and adapting. It requires ongoing research, exploring new information, and being open to adjusting your habits as needed.

Embrace the challenge, stay curious, and enjoy the process of discovering what truly nourishes your body and mind. Remember, there is no single "right" way to eat.

By listening to your body, experimenting with different foods and lifestyle changes, and staying informed about the latest research, you can empower yourself to make informed choices and thrive on a path towards optimal health and longevity.

CHAPTER 6: BEYOND THE PYRAMID: EMBRACING THE DIET FOR OPTIMAL HEALTH

For decades, dietary guidelines like the Food Pyramid have steered the public towards a processed, carbohydrate-heavy diet that includes an excess of high-saturated-fat animal products, ultimately contributing to a rise in obesity, cancer, diabetes and heart disease.

As we move forward into a new era of understanding about the human body and its relationship with food, a compelling case emerges for embracing a raw plant-based diet as the most natural and beneficial approach to optimal health and longevity.

This chapter delves into the scientific evidence and compelling arguments that support the raw plant-based lifestyle.

Reconnecting with Our Ancestral Roots

From an evolutionary perspective, our bodies are finely tuned to a plant-based diet. Research suggests that our ancestors thrived for millions of years on a diet rich in raw fruits, leafy greens, vegetables, nuts, and seeds, readily available in their natural environment. This ancestral dietary pattern provided a balanced source of essential nutrients and fiber, promoting optimal health and survival.

Dr. Milton Mills, author of "The Primal Diet," emphasizes that "Our bodies are designed to process and extract nutrients from plants. However, the abundance of processed foods, animal products and refined sugars in our modern diet is a recent development, and our bodies haven't fully adapted to these dietary changes."

While humans developed the ability to consume cooked food later in evolution, processed foods, refined sugars, and excessive amounts of animal products are modern inventions that our bodies haven't fully adapted to.

These dietary elements can contribute to inflammation, chronic disease, and ultimately, a shorter lifespan.

Harnessing the Power of Nature's Enzymes

Raw fruits, greens and other vegetables are brimming with vital enzymes essential for digestion and nutrient absorption. Enzymes are nature's catalysts, facilitating the breakdown of food and the efficient extraction of nutrients. Dr. Edward Howell, a pioneer in enzyme research, stated, "Enzymes are the spark plugs of life. Without them, there would be no life."

Cooking, however, destroys these enzymes, placing an additional burden on the digestive system and potentially hindering the body's ability to extract the full benefits from food.

By consuming food in its raw state, we harness the natural power of enzymes, aiding digestion, boosting nutrient absorption, and promoting overall gut health. This can lead to increased energy levels, improved digestion, and a stronger immune system.

The Abundant Power of Plant-Based Nutrients

A raw plant-based diet provides a wealth of essential nutrients, including vitamins, minerals, antioxidants, and fiber. These nutrients play a crucial role in various bodily functions, from supporting cell growth and repair to protecting against chronic diseases.

The National Cancer Institute acknowledges that "Fruits and vegetables are rich in fiber, vitamins, minerals, and other bioactive compounds that may help reduce the risk of chronic diseases, including cancer."

Raw plant-based foods are also naturally low in saturated fat and cholesterol, further promoting a healthy heart and circulatory system. A study published in the Journal of the American Medical Association found that "a plant-based diet can significantly reduce the risk of heart disease, stroke, and type 2 diabetes."

The Detoxifying Power of Raw Food

Raw fruits and vegetables are nature's detoxifiers, containing compounds that help cleanse the body of harmful toxins and waste products. These compounds work by stimulating the liver, promoting the elimination of toxins through the digestive system, and enhancing the body's natural detoxification processes.

Dr. Ann Wigmore, renowned author and founder of the Hippocrates Health Institute, believed that "The raw food diet is the most effective way to detoxify the body and restore health."

By eliminating processed foods and animal products, which can contribute to inflammation and toxin buildup, a raw plant-based diet allows the body's natural detoxification processes to function optimally, leading to a cleaner and healthier internal environment.

Beyond the Physical Benefits: A Holistic Approach to Well-being

The benefits of a raw plant-based diet extend beyond the physical realm. Embracing this lifestyle can foster a deeper connection with nature, promoting a sense of awareness and appreciation for the Earth's bounty. The alignment with natural cycles and the act of consuming food directly from the source can bring a sense of mindfulness and peace to the eating experience.

Additionally, the ethical implications of animal agriculture often resonate with individuals who choose a raw vegan path. By embracing a lifestyle that avoids animal exploitation, individuals can align their dietary choices with their values and contribute to a more compassionate and sustainable world.

Moving Beyond the Pyramid: A Roadmap to Optimal Health

The Food Pyramid, with its flawed recommendations and biased influences, has led many astray from the path of optimal health. By embracing a raw plant-based diet, individuals can reconnect with their ancestral roots, harness the power of nature's bounty, and take the next steps toward optimal health, well-being, and alignment with their values.

Remember, the path towards a raw plant-based lifestyle is a gradual process requiring commitment and exploration. By seeking guidance from qualified professionals, experimenting with different raw food recipes, and embracing a mindful approach to eating, individuals can discover a vibrant and fulfilling life fueled by the power of raw, plant-based nutrition.

Steps to a Healthier Dietary Lifestyle

Here are some key steps to begin your new raw plant-based lifestyle:

1. Education and Research: Immerse yourself in the science and philosophy behind raw foodism. Read books and articles by experts like Dr. Douglas Graham, Dr. Gabriel Cousens, Victoria Boutenko and myself, Alice Dee. Watch documentaries like "Forks Over Knives" and "Fat, Sick & Nearly Dead" to gain inspiration and learn from others' experiences.

2. Gradual Transition: Start slowly by incorporating more raw fruits and vegetables into your diet. Replace processed snacks with raw versions like fruit slices, nuts, and seeds. Gradually increase the percentage of raw foods in your meals, allowing your body time to adjust.

3. Culinary Exploration: Discover the joy of raw food preparation. Experiment with different recipes for smoothies, salads, soups, and main courses. Explore resources like "The Complete Book of Raw Food" by Brenda Davis and "Raw Food for Beginners" by Kristina Carrillo-Bucaram for delicious and easy-to-follow recipes.

4. Community Connection: Seek out support and guidance from a community of raw food enthusiasts. Join online forums, attend workshops and retreats, and connect with local raw food groups. Sharing your experience with others can provide valuable insights, motivation, and a sense of belonging.

5. Mindful Eating: Cultivate a mindful approach to eating. Focus on the taste, texture, and aroma of your food, savoring each bite and appreciating the natural nourishment it provides. Disconnect from distractions and prioritize the act of eating, allowing your body to fully absorb the nutrients and experience the joy of mindful nourishment.

6. Listen to Your Body: Pay close attention to your body's signals. Observe how different raw foods make you feel, identifying what works best for your unique needs and preferences. Adjust your diet accordingly; honoring your body's wisdom and making conscious choices that support your overall well-being.

7. Embrace the Transition: Remember, transitioning to a raw plant-based lifestyle is a path, not a destination. There will be challenges and setbacks along the way, but don't get discouraged. Celebrate your successes, learn from your experiences, and enjoy the process of discovering a healthier, happier, and more fulfilling way of life.

By embracing a raw plant-based diet and taking these steps, you can embark on a path towards optimal health, reconnect with your natural essence, and experience the vibrant energy and vitality that comes from nurturing your body with the raw power of the natural diet you were born to consume.

CHAPTER 7: THE PROCESSED FOOD LABYRINTH: DECODING THE INGREDIENTS LIST

In today's fast-paced world, processed foods often beckon with their convenience and apparent affordability. Yet, lurking beneath the glossy packaging and enticing marketing slogans lies a hidden labyrinth of ingredients, many of which can pose a significant threat to our health and well-being.

This chapter delves into the murky depths of the processed food industry, providing individuals with the knowledge and tools to navigate the complex world of food labels and make informed dietary choices that support optimal health.

Understanding Common Food Additives and Their Hidden Dangers

Processed foods are often laden with a plethora of additives, designed to enhance flavor, texture, shelf life, and appearance. While some additives may be deemed safe in limited amounts, many pose serious health risks, contributing to a range of chronic diseases, including:

- **Artificial sweeteners:** Aspartame, sucralose, and saccharin, commonly found in diet sodas and processed snacks, have been linked to cancer, obesity, and metabolic disorders. The National Cancer Institute acknowledges that "studies suggest a potential link between artificial sweeteners and an increased risk of cancer."

- **Preservatives:** Sodium benzoate, potassium sorbate, and nitrates, used to extend shelf life, can disrupt gut bacteria and potentially contribute to inflammatory bowel disease and other health problems. Dr. Michael Greger, author of "How Not to Die," emphasizes that "Preservatives may be harmful to gut bacteria, which play a crucial role in overall health."

- **Emulsifiers:** Polysorbate 80 and carrageenan, common thickeners and stabilizers, have been linked to digestive issues, inflammation, and even colon cancer. A study published in the journal "Nature" found that "carrageenan can cause intestinal inflammation and promote tumor growth in animal models."

- **Artificial colors and flavors:** These additives, often derived from petroleum or other synthetic sources, can trigger allergic reactions, hyperactivity, and even behavioral problems in children. The Center for Science in the Public Interest warns that "artificial food dyes can be harmful to children's health, causing hyperactivity and behavioral problems."

How to Read Labels Like a Pro

Navigating the labyrinth of processed food labels requires a keen eye and a thorough understanding of key ingredients. Here are some essential tips to decode the cryptic language and make informed choices:

1. Read the entire ingredients list: Don't just focus on the front of the packaging. Turn the product over and carefully read the ingredients list, paying particular attention to the first few ingredients, as they are listed in descending order of quantity.

2. Decode hidden names: Many unhealthy ingredients are disguised under confusing or seemingly innocuous names. Familiarize yourself with common aliases, such as "hydrolyzed vegetable protein" (often a source of gluten and MSG) and "carrageenan" (often listed as "seaweed extract").

3. Prioritize whole plant foods: Choose products with a short and recognizable ingredients list, predominantly consisting of whole foods like fruits, vegetables, whole grains, and nuts. Avoid foods that come from animals including meat, milk, butter, eggs, gelatin and lard.

4. Avoid artificial additives: Look for products free of artificial sweeteners, colors, flavors, and preservatives. Opt for natural alternatives like stevia for sweetness, turmeric for color, and herbs and spices for flavor.

5. Be mindful of serving sizes: Pay close attention to serving sizes listed on the label. Often, the suggested serving size is significantly smaller than the actual amount consumed, leading to overconsumption of calories and unhealthy ingredients.

6. Keep salt content low: If you have issues with high blood pressure, avoid processed foods that contain salt. You can often look at labels to see the sodium content of foods.

Avoiding Processed Foods and Creating a Healthy Kitchen

Empowering yourself with label-reading skills is just the first step. To truly escape the processed food labyrinth, it's crucial to shift your focus towards whole, unprocessed foods and cultivate a healthy kitchen environment. Here are some practical strategies:

1. Plan your meals: Take time each week to plan your meals and snacks. This allows you to make conscious choices about the ingredients you consume and avoid the temptation of grabbing processed quick fixes.

2. Stock your pantry with healthy staples: Keep your pantry stocked with whole grains, legumes, nuts, seeds, dried fruits, and spices. These versatile ingredients provide the foundation for creating delicious and nutritious meals at home.

3. Invest in fresh produce: Prioritize fresh fruits, leafy greens and other vegetables whenever possible. Explore farmer's markets and local grocery stores to find seasonal produce at its peak flavor and nutritional value. Consider choosing organic and planting a food forest to grow your own produce.

4. Embrace simple dishes: Preparing food doesn't have to be complicated. Explore simple recipes that utilize whole, raw plant-derived ingredients and require minimal preparation time. Master basic preparation techniques like blending, dehydrating, food processing, grinding, and chopping to unlock a world of culinary possibilities.

5. Make it a family affair: Involve your family in meal planning and preparation. This fosters a sense of ownership and encourages healthy eating habits for everyone.

Breaking Free from the Labyrinth: Embracing a Whole Food Lifestyle

Breaking free from the processed and cooked food labyrinth requires vigilance, awareness, and a commitment to nourishing your body with whole, unprocessed and raw plant foods.

By understanding the hidden dangers of common additives, learning to decipher food labels, and embracing a whole food plant-based kitchen, individuals can empower themselves to make informed dietary choices and navigate the often-confusing world of food.

Beyond Label Reading: Cultivating a Holistic Approach to Food

Focusing solely on label reading can sometimes feel restrictive and overwhelming. While understanding food labels is important, it's equally vital to cultivate a holistic approach to food that extends beyond simply avoiding unhealthy ingredients. Here are some additional strategies for embracing a whole food lifestyle:

1. **Mindfulness and Gratitude:** Approach your meals with mindfulness and gratitude. Savor each bite, appreciate the natural flavors and textures of your food, and be thankful for the nourishment it provides. This conscious approach can enhance your relationship with food and promote mindful eating habits.

2. **Culinary Creativity:** Explore the world of preparing whole and raw plant-based foods with creativity and joy. Experiment with different recipes, discover new flavors, and find ways to incorporate a variety of fruits, greens, vegetables, whole grains, nuts, seeds, and legumes into your meals.

3. **Building a Support System:** Surround yourself with others who share your passion for healthy eating. Join cooking groups, attend workshops, and connect with individuals who can provide encouragement and support for your process.

4. **Embracing the Imperfections:** Remember, progress, not perfection, is key. There will be days when convenience wins and processed foods sneak into your diet. Don't be discouraged by occasional setbacks. Acknowledge them, learn from them, and recommit to your whole-food goals.

5. Prioritizing Personal Well-Being: Remember that food is just one piece of the puzzle when it comes to optimal health. Combine a whole-food plant-based diet with regular physical activity, stress management techniques, and adequate sleep to truly thrive.

Embracing a whole food, raw plant-based lifestyle is not about deprivation or fad diets. It's about making conscious choices that nourish your body, mind, and soul.

By venturing beyond the processed food labyrinth and embracing the abundance of whole, unprocessed and raw plant foods, you can unlock the door to a healthier, happier, and more fulfilling life.

Remember, the path towards a whole food lifestyle is a lifelong process, filled with learning, exploration, and joy. Embrace the adventure, savor the deliciousness of real food suitable for your species, and empower yourself to make informed choices that support your well-being.

By incorporating the information from resources like this book into your lifestyle, you can equip yourself with the knowledge and tools to navigate the complex food landscape and cultivate a vibrant life fueled by the power of whole, unprocessed and raw plant-based nourishment.

CHAPTER 8: THE MEAT MYTH: EXPOSING THE ENVIRONMENTAL AND HEALTH COSTS OF ANIMAL AGRICULTURE

For generations, meat has been lauded as a dietary pillar, ingrained in cultural traditions and portrayed as a symbol of strength and vitality.

However, beneath this facade lies a stark reality: animal agriculture, the process of raising and slaughtering animals for food, poses a significant threat to our planet and can be devastating to our health.

This chapter delves into the unsettling truth behind the meat myth, exposing its devastating environmental impact, the growing dangers of antibiotic resistance, and unveiling healthier and more sustainable alternatives that promote both individual well-being and planetary health.

The Looming Shadow of Animal Agriculture on Climate Change

The livestock industry is a major contributor to climate change, accounting for approximately 14.5% of global greenhouse gas emissions. Livestock produce methane, a potent greenhouse gas with 86 times the warming potential of carbon dioxide over a 20-year period.

In addition, animal agriculture contributes to deforestation, as vast land areas are cleared to support grazing and feed production, leading to a loss of vital carbon sinks.

The United Nations Food and Agriculture Organization (FAO) acknowledges that "Animal agriculture is one of the leading causes of deforestation, global warming, and water pollution."

The sheer volume of resources consumed by animal agriculture further amplifies its environmental footprint. Raising livestock requires vast quantities of water, with an estimated 2,400 gallons of water needed to produce just one pound of beef. This unsustainable water usage strains limited resources and contributes to water scarcity in many regions.

The Growing Threat of Antibiotic Resistance and Factory Farming

Factory farms, where animals are densely confined in unsanitary conditions, have become breeding grounds for antibiotic-resistant bacteria. The overuse of antibiotics in livestock farming to prevent illness and promote growth creates a selective environment where resistant bacteria thrive and spread.

The World Health Organization (WHO) warns that "Antibiotic resistance is one of the biggest threats to global health, food security, and development."

Antibiotic-resistant bacteria can infect humans through the food chain, causing potentially deadly infections that are increasingly difficult to treat. This growing public health threat underscores the urgent need to transition away from intensive animal agriculture practices.

Beyond the Plate: The Ethical Implications of Meat Consumption

The production of meat inherently involves the suffering and exploitation of sentient beings. Animals raised for food are subjected to inhumane conditions, including confinement, forced breeding, and painful procedures.

This raises significant ethical concerns regarding the treatment of sentient beings and the potential for inflicting unnecessary suffering. Moreover, the slaughter of animals involves immense pain and distress, sparking ethical debates about the morality of consuming meat and the potential for building a more compassionate food system.

Healthier and More Sustainable Alternatives to Meat

The good news is that a growing body of evidence highlights the numerous advantages of adopting a plant-based diet. Research suggests that a plant-based diet can significantly reduce the risk of chronic diseases such as heart disease, obesity, type 2 diabetes, high blood pressure, and certain cancers.

Keep in mind that The American Heart Association acknowledges that "A well-planned plant-based diet can be a healthy and sustainable way to meet your nutritional needs."

Furthermore, plant-based diets are typically lower in saturated fat and cholesterol, contributing to a healthier heart and overall cardiovascular system. Additionally, plant-based diets offer a wealth of essential nutrients, including vitamins, minerals, fiber, and antioxidants, vital for optimal health and well-being.

Embarking on a Path of Compassion and Sustainability

Transitioning towards a plant-based diet is not just about personal health; it's also a powerful act of compassion and environmental responsibility. By choosing a plant-based lifestyle, individuals contribute to mitigating climate change, reducing their carbon footprint, and protecting valuable resources.

Moreover, choosing a plant-based diet aligns with ethical values that promote compassion for all living beings and respect for the natural world. This holistic approach to food can foster a sense of deeper connection with the environment and contribute to a more sustainable future for all.

The Meat Myth: A Call to Action

The unsettling truth about the environmental and health costs of animal agriculture demands a critical reevaluation of our dietary choices. By embracing a raw, whole food, plant-based diet, individuals can empower themselves to protect their health, safeguard the planet, and align their values with a more compassionate and sustainable future.

The path towards a plant-based lifestyle is filled with delicious discoveries, vibrant flavors, and a sense of empowerment that comes with taking control of your health and contributing to a better world.

By embracing the abundance of plant-based foods and exploring resources like "The China Study" by T. Colin Campbell and "Forks Over Knives" by Dr. John McDougall, as well as other books and resources from this author, individuals can embark on a path towards optimal health, ecological sustainability, and a life filled with compassion for all living beings.

Remember, your dietary choices hold immense power. By making informed decisions and choosing a plant-based diet, you can become a force for positive change

Here are some additional steps to make the transition to a plant-based diet:

- **Start gradually:** Don't try to change everything overnight. Begin by incorporating more plant-based meals into your week, gradually increasing your intake over time.

- **Experiment with different flavors and recipes:** Explore the vast world of plant-based cuisine. Discover new fruits, vegetables, nuts, seeds, and grains to create delicious and nutritious meals.

- **Seek support:** Connect with others who have transitioned to a plant-based diet. Share experiences, recipes, and encouragement to support each other on your personal paths.

- **Listen to your body:** Pay attention to how you feel after consuming different foods. Choose plant-based options that make you feel energized, satisfied, and healthy.

- **Embrace the path:** Remember, transitioning to a plant-based diet is a process, not a destination. Celebrate your victories, learn from your experiences, and enjoy the delicious and rewarding path towards optimal health and well-being.

By embracing a plant-based lifestyle, you are not only nourishing your body, but also taking a stand for a healthier planet, greater compassion for all living beings, and a more sustainable future for generations to come.

Remember, the future of our planet and our health lies in the choices we make today. Choose plant-based, choose compassion, and choose a brighter future for all.

CONCLUSION: DO RESEARCH, RECLAIM YOUR HEALTH, AND FIGHT BACK AGAINST THE DIETARY CONSPIRACY

In the face of a government-subsidized food system heavily influenced by corporate interests that prioritize profits over public health and covert public policies aimed at increasing the risk of an early death for retirees, the responsibility for our well-being ultimately rests in our own hands.

By embracing a raw, whole-food, plant-based diet, we can reclaim control over our health, fight back against the human dietary conspiracy our government does not want us to recognize, and pave the way for a brighter future for ourselves, our children, our communities, and the planet.

Practical Tips for Creating Better Health by Hacking the Dietary System

Learning how to live a raw plant-based lifestyle requires commitment and action. Here are some practical tips to guide you:

- **Start small:** Don't feel pressured to make drastic changes overnight. Introduce plant-based meals gradually, replacing one processed food at a time with whole, unprocessed alternatives.

- **Explore the rainbow:** Embrace the abundance of fruits. greens and other vegetables available in diverse colors. Each color offers unique nutrients and contributes to a balanced diet.

- **Embrace diversity:** Experiment with different plant-based protein sources like sprouted legumes and grains, as well as soaked nuts and seeds to ensure your raw plant-powered diet provides all essential amino acids.

- **Prepare food more often:** Discover the joy and health benefits of preparing raw whole foods at home. This allows you to control ingredients and create delicious, nutritious meals that align with your healthier dietary preferences.

- **Plan and prepare:** Planning your meals and snacks in advance can help you avoid unhealthy temptations and ensure you have healthy options readily available.

Research Resources and Tools for Sustainable Eating

Fortunately, numerous resources and tools can empower you in your raw plant-based lifestyle:

- **Books:** "The Nutritional Healer" by Alice Dee, "The China Study" by T. Colin Campbell, "Forks Over Knives" by Dr. John McDougall, and "The Starch Solution" by Dr. John McDougall.

- **Websites:** Forks Over Knives, Raw From the Garden, The Plantrician Project, and Happy Herbivore.

- **Documentaries:** Forks Over Knives, Fat, Sick & Nearly Dead, The Game Changers, and What the Health.

- **Apps:** Cronometer, HappyCow, Mealime

- **Community:** Join supportive online forums like Facebook Groups, attend local events, and connect with other plant-based individuals to share experiences and get support from like-minded people.

Good News from the American Dietetic Association

The American Dietetic Association (ADA, now known as the Academy of Nutrition and Dietetics) is one of the largest professional organizations in the world. It officially recognizes plant-based (vegan) diets as healthy, nutritionally adequate, and potentially beneficial in the prevention and treatment of certain chronic diseases. Here's a summary of their position:

Overall Position:

- Plant-based diets, including vegan and vegetarian diets, can be healthful and nutritionally adequate for all stages of the life cycle, including pregnancy, lactation, infancy, childhood, and adolescence, and for athletes.

- Well-planned plant-based diets can provide all the nutrients needed for good health.

- Plant-based diets may offer protection against several chronic diseases, including heart disease, obesity, type 2 diabetes, and some types of cancer.

Specifics:

- Vegan diets require careful planning to ensure adequate intake of essential nutrients, particularly vitamin B12, vitamin D, omega-3 fatty acids, iron, calcium, and zinc.

- Vegetarian diets offer more flexibility, but it's still important to be mindful of nutrient intake. They tend to have a higher saturated fat intake, however.

- Individuals transitioning to a plant-based diet should consult with a registered dietitian, plant-based nutritionist, or other qualified healthcare professional to help them create a safe and effective plan.

Resources and Position Papers:

- Official website of the ADA (now the Academy of Nutrition and Dietetics): https://www.eatright.org/

- Position of the Academy of Nutrition and Dietetics: Vegetarian Diets

- Academy of Nutrition and Dietetics: Plant-Based Diets

In addition, the ADA has published several other resources on plant-based diets, including:

- Vegetarian Nutrition

- Plant-Based Protein

- Iron in Plant-Based Diets

- Calcium in Plant-Based Diets

Overall, the American Dietetic Association strongly supports plant-based diets as a healthy and sustainable way of eating for all people.

A Brighter Future for Food, Health, and Enjoying a Long Retirement

By choosing a raw, whole-food, plant-based diet, you are not only investing in your immediate health but also contributing to a brighter futureyou're your retirement and for generations to come. Here are just a few of the benefits you can expect:

- **Improved health:** Reduced risk of chronic diseases like heart disease, obesity, type II diabetes, and certain cancers, while enjoying increased energy levels and improved digestion.

- **Enhanced vitality:** Feel lighter, stronger, and more energized as you nourish your body with natural, unprocessed foods.

- **Sustainable living:** Reduce your carbon footprint, conserve valuable resources, and contribute to a more sustainable food system.

- **Ethical alignment:** Choose a lifestyle that aligns with your values of compassion for all living beings.

- **Long and healthy retirement:** Enjoy a long, active retirement free from the burden of chronic diseases, allowing you to live life to the fullest.

Remember, the choice to reclaim your health and fight back against the dietary conspiracy is yours. By embracing a raw, whole-food, plant-based diet, you can unlock a world of vibrant health, contribute to a sustainable future, and experience the joy of a life fueled by the power of real, unprocessed food.

Together, we can create a world where healthy, sustainable food choices are readily available and accessible to all. Keep in mind that you are not alone on this healthier path. A growing community of individuals committed to a plant-based lifestyle exists, and we stand ready to support and empower you every step of the way.

Start today by choosing raw plant-based whole foods so you can reclaim your health and enjoy a brighter and more fulfilling retirement and planetary future for coming generations.

Reclaiming Your Health and Rising Up Against the Dietary Deception

In the face of the seemingly insurmountable challenge of a massive government-subsidized food system tightly woven with corporate interests, we stand at a pivotal point in history. This food system, driven by profit and concern over dwindling retirement fund resources, operates at the expense of public health by actively promoting unhealthy dietary choices that subtly undermine our well-being and shorten our lifespans, if not detected and countered in time.

This veiled dietary conspiracy, hidden behind layers of misinformation and heavily manipulated scientific research, clearly seeks to maintain the current power structure, boost corporate profits and eliminate taxpayers shortly after their retirement, thereby leaving the human population vulnerable to chronic diseases and a premature demise.

Amidst this seemingly bleak landscape, however, hope still blooms. The power to reclaim our health and overturn this insidious and deceptive food conspiracy lies within our own hands. By embracing a raw, whole-food, plant-based diet, we can rise up against this deception, hack the retirement system, and rewrite the script for ourselves, our loved ones, and future generations.

Keep in mind that choosing a plant-based lifestyle is not just about individual health; it's a rebellion against the secret government plot to send you to an early grave after you have dutifully paid taxes all your working life. It is an essential act of defiance against a devious public system that drains money derived from your hard work and then benefits from facilitating your early demise. It also takes a firm stand against the greedy people who run corporations that profit from your ailments and thrive on your dietary ignorance.

By rejecting the processed foods and animal-based products they aim to push down our innocently unsuspecting throats, we can break free from their control and reclaim the power to nourish our bodies with the vibrant energy of nature's bounty. We can invest in our retirements and gain the cherished ability to live long, healthy lives as we were born to do.

This path is not without its challenges, however. We must learn to confidently navigate a world saturated with conflicting information, misleading advertisements, and deeply ingrained cultural habits and traditions. We need to buck prevailing dietary trends, forgo eating at the greedy fast food restaurants, and avoid unhealthy animal products, sugary drinks, and processed snacks. Happily, the rewards in terms of our better health and longevity well into our golden retirement years remain immeasurable.

By embracing a raw, plant-based lifestyle, we unlock a world of vibrant health, boundless energy, and increased vitality. We become empowered to take control of our well-being, prevent and even reverse chronic diseases, and pave the way for a long and fulfilling life where we can act as reservoirs of wisdom for our children, grandchildren and society in general.

Furthermore, the benefits of this lifestyle extend far beyond our individual well-being. By choosing a plant-based lifestyle, we contribute to a more sustainable future for our planet.

We also reduce our carbon footprint, conserve precious resources, and protect the environment for generations to come. Finally, we align ourselves with the universal values of compassion and ethical treatment of all living beings, creating a ripple effect of positive change throughout the world consistent with the Golden Rule.

Moving Forward on the Right Dietary Path

Let this book be your call to action. Hear its clarion call to see into and rise above the dietary deception your government and big corporations want you to swallow so you can embrace a brighter future for yourself, your offspring, other living beings, and your planet.

Let us henceforth vow to nourish our bodies only with the wisdom of nature, rejecting the unhealthy processed and animal-derived food products that have long been erroneously held up as dietary pillars. Let us lead by our example as we become beacons of health and vitality, inspiring others to join us in this process of transformation.

Together, we can break the chains of the human dietary conspiracy and build a new world, one where healthy, sustainable, plant-based food choices are readily available and accessible to all. Let us show our government that we see through their veiled agenda and choose health, well-being, a long retirement, and a vibrant future for ourselves and the planet.

The time for action is now! Embark on your plant-based path today. Reclaim your health, fight back against the dietary deception, and join the uprising against devious government food subsidy practices for a brighter tomorrow.

53

APPENDICES

APPENDIX A: ADDITIONAL RESOURCES AND FURTHER READING

To help you further your research into the topics addressed in this book, this appendix contains a list of additional resources and further readings. Please note that this is not an exhaustive list, and there are many other valuable resources available on the topic of plant-based eating and healthy living. The best resources for you will depend on your individual needs and preferences. As always, do your own research and find what works best for you.

Books:

- Forks Over Knives: The Plant-Based Way to Health by T. Colin Campbell, M.D., and Caldwell B. Esselstyn, Jr., M.D.
- The China Study: The Most Comprehensive Study of Nutrition Ever Conducted and the Startling Implications for Diet, Weight Loss, and Long-Term Health by T. Colin Campbell, Ph.D., and Thomas M. Campbell II, M.D.
- The Nutritional Healer: Creating Wellness with Better Food Choices by Alice Dee.
- The Starch Solution: Eat the Foods You Love, Regain Your Health, and Lose the Weight for Good by John McDougall, M.D.
- The Processed Food Trap: How Food Companies Exploit Your Brain and Control Your Eating Habits by Stephanie Cacioppo, Ph.D., and John Cacioppo, Ph.D.
- The Grain Brain: The Surprising Truth about Wheat, Carbs, and Sugar - Your Brain's Silent Killers by David Perlmutter, M.D.
- The Meat Myth: Why Animal Protein Is Making You Sick and What You Can Do About It by David Robinson Simon.
- Why Vegan? Reasons to Boycott Animal Use by Alice Dee.
- Eating Animals: A Moral Investigation by Jonathan Safran Foer.
- Animal Liberation: The Definitive Classic of Animal Rights and Veganism by Peter Singer.
- The Food Forest Guide: How to Cultivate an Edible Landscape for

Good Health and Harvests by Alice Dee.
- Raw Vegan Recipes by Alice Dee.

Websites:

- Forks Over Knives: https://www.forksoverknives.com/
- Raw From the Garden: http://RawFromTheGarden.com
- The Plantrician Project: https://plantricianproject.org/
- Happy Herbivore: https://happyherbivore.com/
- NutritionFacts.org: https://nutritionfacts.org/
- The Vegan Society: https://www.vegansociety.com/
- The Environmental Working Group: https://www.ewg.org/
- The Good Food Institute: https://gfi.org/

Documentaries:

- Forks Over Knives
- Fat, Sick & Nearly Dead
- What the Health
- The Game Changers
- Cowspiracy
- Earthlings
- Dominion

Apps:

- Cronometer: https://cronometer.com/
- HappyCow: https://www.happycow.net/search
- Mealime: https://www.mealime.com/

Other Resources:

- American Dietetic Association: https://www.eatright.org/
- Physicians Committee for Responsible Medicine: https://www.pcrm.org/
- We Care About Animals: http://www.WeCareAboutAnimals.org
- The Humane Society of the United States: https://www.humanesociety.org/

APPENDIX B: GLOSSARY OF TERMS

Below you will find a glossary of terms for "The Human Dietary Conspiracy" that you might find useful to understand.

Additives: Substances added to food to improve flavor, texture, color, shelf life, or other properties. Some common additives are sugar, salt, artificial sweeteners, preservatives, and coloring agents.

Animal Agriculture: The practice of raising and breeding animals for food, fiber, and other products.

Biofortification: The process of breeding crops to increase their nutrient content.

Calorie: A unit of energy used to measure the energy content of food.

Carbohydrates: One of the three macronutrients (along with protein and fat) that provide the body with energy. Carbohydrates are found in starchy foods like grains, legumes, fruits, and vegetables.

Cholesterol: A waxy, fat-like substance found in all animal cells and produced by the liver. High levels of LDL ("bad") cholesterol can increase the risk of heart disease. Only animal foods contain cholesterol.

Chronic disease: A long-term illness that cannot be cured, but can often be managed with lifestyle changes and medication. Examples of chronic diseases include heart disease, diabetes, cancer, and Alzheimer's disease.

Detoxification: The process of removing harmful toxins from the body.

Ethical veganism: A philosophy and lifestyle that rejects the exploitation of animals for food, clothing, or any other purpose whenever possible and practical.

Factory farming: An intensive method of raising animals in large, confined spaces.

Fiber: A type of carbohydrate that the body cannot digest. Fiber helps to keep the digestive system healthy and can lower cholesterol levels.

Gluten: A protein found in wheat, barley, and rye. Gluten can cause digestive problems for people with celiac disease and gluten sensitivity.

GMO (genetically modified organism): An organism that has had its genetic makeup altered in a way that does not occur naturally.

Industrial agriculture: A large-scale, intensive system of farming that relies on monoculture, chemical fertilizers and pesticides, and genetic engineering.

Longevity: The length of time that a person lives.

Macronutrients: Nutrients that the body needs in large amounts, including carbohydrates, protein, and fat.

Micronutrients: Nutrients that the body needs in small amounts, including vitamins and minerals.

Processed food: Food that has been altered from its natural state through processing, such as canning, freezing, cooking, or adding preservatives.

Refined grains: Grains that have had the bran and germ removed, leaving behind the starchy endosperm. Refined grains are less nutritious than whole grains.

Saturated fat: A type of fat that is solid at room temperature. Saturated fat is found in animal products and some plant-based foods, such as coconut oil, palm oil, and hydrogenated vegetable oil.

Social Security: A government program that provides financial assistance to retirees, disabled individuals, and survivors of deceased workers.

Subsidy: A financial payment made by the government to a producer or consumer of a product or service.

Sugar addiction: A condition in which a person has a strong craving for sugar and experiences withdrawal symptoms when they try to cut back.

Sustainable agriculture: A farming system that meets the needs of the present without compromising the ability of future generations to meet their own needs.

Unprocessed food: Food in its natural state, such as fruits, leafy greens, other vegetables, whole grains, legumes, nuts, and seeds.

Vegan: A person who does not engage in exploiting or killing animals for ethical reasons. Vegans do not eat any animal products, including meat, dairy, eggs, and honey.

Whole grains: Grains that contain all of their original parts - the bran, germ, and endosperm. Whole grains are more nutritious and natural than refined grains.

ABOUT THE AUTHOR

After obtaining her physical science degrees, Alice Dee then studied nutritional healing and herbology for decades. In addition to growing a thriving food forest, Alice also founded a pioneering raw plant-based restaurant in Northern California. Alice is the author of several other books related to plant-based diets, as well as the organizer of related online forums. Alice is currently available for speaking engagements regarding the Human Dietary Conspiracy, as well as for consulting on nutritional healing and plant-based diets. For more information, please visit her websites at:

www.HumanDietaryConspiracy.com

www.PeakPerformanceDiet.com

www.TheFoodForestGuide.com

www.NutritionalHealer.com

www.RawFromTheGarden.com

For fully raw plant-based recipes you can make to support your return to better health so you can enjoy a long retirement, you can buy Alice's restaurant-tested Raw Vegan Recipes book here:

www.RawVeganRecipesBook.com

For additional support, you can join her large and active Raw Vegan Recipes Facebook Group here:

www.facebook.com/groups/rawveganrecipes1/